FLORIDAX WITH IRON

A Plant Based Approach for Prevention of Iron Deficiency in Pregnant Women and Children

Selena Curtis

Table of Contents

Introduction

In a world teeming with technological advancements and medical breakthroughs, it's a startling paradox that one of the most abundant elements on Earth continues to elude the grasp of human biology. Iron, the very foundation of our planet's core, the building block of industrial revolutions, and a critical component of life itself, remains frustratingly scarce within the bodies of millions. This scarcity, particularly prevalent among pregnant women and children, paints a somber picture of a global health crisis hiding in plain sight.

As you embark on this journey through the pages of "Floridax with Iron: A Plant Based Approach for Prevention of Iron Deficiency in Pregnant Women and Children," prepare to unravel the complexities of this paradox and discover a groundbreaking solution rooted in the wisdom of nature itself.

Iron deficiency, often dubbed the "silent epidemic," affects an estimated two billion people worldwide. It's a staggering figure that belies the element's ubiquity in our environment. Yet, for pregnant women nurturing new life within them and children laying the foundations for their future, this deficiency can cast long shadows over their health and potential.

Imagine a young mother-to-be, her body working tirelessly to support not just one, but two lives. Her need for iron skyrockets, sometimes doubling or even tripling. Without adequate iron, she faces increased risks of premature birth, low birth weight, and postpartum depression. The child within her, dependent on her resources, may enter the world already at a disadvantage, potentially facing cognitive delays and weakened immunity.

Now picture a vibrant young child, full of curiosity and promise. Iron deficiency can dim that spark, sapping energy, impairing cognitive development, and stunting physical growth. The consequences ripple outward, affecting academic performance, social interactions, and ultimately, life opportunities.

These scenarios are not mere hypotheticals but daily realities for millions. The traditional approach to addressing this crisis has relied heavily on synthetic iron supplements. While these have their place, they often come with a host of side effects – nausea, constipation, metallic taste – leading to poor compliance and limited effectiveness. It's a bitter pill to swallow, quite literally, for those already grappling with the challenges of pregnancy or childhood nutrition.

But what if there was another way? What if the solution to this modern health crisis lay not in laboratories and factories, but in the lush diversity of the plant kingdom?

Enter Floridax – a revolutionary plant-based iron supplement that promises to bridge the gap between nature's abundance and our body's needs. Derived from a carefully curated blend of iron-rich botanicals, Floridax represents a paradigm shift in how we approach iron supplementation.

The story of Floridax is one of innovation rooted in ancient wisdom. For millennia, cultures around the world have turned to specific plants known for their iron content. From the mineral-rich herbs of Traditional Chinese Medicine to the iron-packed greens favored in African cuisines, this knowledge has been passed down through generations. Floridax harnesses these time-tested botanical sources, combining them with cutting-edge extraction techniques to create a supplement that's both potent and bioavailable.

But Floridax is more than just a supplement; it's a philosophy. It embodies a return to nature, a recognition that sometimes the best solutions are those that have been growing around us all along. In a world increasingly disconnected from its natural roots, Floridax serves as a reminder of the power and wisdom inherent in the plant kingdom.

As we journey deeper into the pages of this book, we'll explore the science behind Floridax, unraveling how this plant-based formula can outperform traditional iron supplements in bioavailability and tolerability. We'll examine clinical studies that demonstrate its efficacy in pregnant women and children, and discover how its benefits extend beyond mere iron supplementation.

You'll learn about the synergistic blend of botanicals that make up Floridax, each chosen not just for its iron content, but for the array of complementary nutrients it provides. This holistic approach sets Floridax apart, offering a more complete nutritional profile that supports overall health and well-being.

We'll also address the practical aspects of incorporating Floridax into daily life. From pregnancy to childhood and beyond, you'll find guidance on dosages, usage, and potential interactions. Real-life success stories will illustrate the transformative potential of this natural approach, painting vivid pictures of renewed energy, improved cognitive function, and strengthened immunity.

But this book isn't just about Floridax. It's a comprehensive guide to understanding and addressing iron deficiency through a plant-based lens. We'll explore iron-rich meal plans, clever food combinations that enhance absorption, and lifestyle factors that influence iron status. This holistic approach empowers you to take control of your iron health, with Floridax as a powerful ally in your journey.

In the pages that follow, prepare to challenge your assumptions about iron supplementation. Whether you're an expectant mother, a parent concerned about your child's development, a healthcare practitioner seeking alternative approaches, or simply someone interested in natural health solutions, this book offers valuable insights and practical strategies.

Chapter 1

The Silent Epidemic - Understanding Iron Deficiency

In the spectrum of human health, iron stands out as a thread of paramount importance, weaving its way through every cell and system in our bodies. Yet, despite its crucial role, iron deficiency has become a silent epidemic, affecting billions worldwide and posing a particular threat to pregnant women and children. As we embark on this exploration of Floridax with Iron, it's essential to first understand the breadth and depth of the challenge we face.

The Essential Element: Iron's Role in Human Health

Iron, the fourth most abundant element in the Earth's crust, plays an indispensable role in human physiology. At its core, iron is a vital component of hemoglobin, the protein in red blood cells responsible for transporting oxygen throughout the body. Without sufficient iron, our cells struggle to receive the oxygen they need to function optimally, leading to a cascade of health issues.

But iron's importance extends far beyond oxygen transport. It's a key player in numerous enzymatic reactions, DNA synthesis, and electron transport in cellular respiration. Iron is crucial for proper brain function, particularly in neurotransmitter synthesis and myelin production. In the immune system, iron helps produce and activate immune cells, forming a critical line of defense against pathogens.

For pregnant women, iron takes on an even more significant role. As the body works to support both mother and developing fetus, iron demands increase dramatically. The growing fetus requires iron for its own development, particularly for brain growth and the formation of its blood supply. Meanwhile, the mother's body increases its own blood volume by up to 50%, necessitating a substantial increase in iron intake.

In children, iron is nothing short of foundational. It supports rapid growth, cognitive development, and the formation of a robust immune system. Iron deficiency in early childhood can have long-lasting effects, potentially impacting academic performance, behavior, and overall health well into adulthood.

Given its myriad crucial functions, one might assume that iron deficiency would be immediately apparent and swiftly addressed. However, the reality is far more complex and concerning.

At-Risk Populations: Pregnant Women and Children

While iron deficiency can affect anyone, certain groups are particularly vulnerable. Pregnant women and children stand at the forefront of this silent epidemic, their increased iron needs often outpacing their intake.

Pregnant Women:

During pregnancy, a woman's iron requirements can increase by up to 50%. This dramatic rise is due to several factors:

1. Increased blood volume: As mentioned earlier, a pregnant woman's blood volume expands significantly to support the growing fetus.

2. Fetal development: The developing baby requires iron for its own growth, particularly in the third trimester when iron stores are built up to support the infant in the first months of life.

3. Placental growth: The placenta, rich in blood vessels, also requires iron for its development.

4. Preparation for blood loss during delivery: The body anticipates blood loss during childbirth and increases iron stores in preparation.

Despite these increased needs, many pregnant women struggle to meet their iron requirements through diet alone. Morning sickness, food aversions, and dietary restrictions can all contribute to inadequate iron intake. Moreover, the common side effects of traditional iron supplements – such as nausea and constipation – can further complicate efforts to maintain adequate iron levels.

Children:

Children, especially in their first years of life, are another group highly susceptible to iron deficiency. Several factors contribute to this vulnerability:

1. Rapid growth: The first three years of life are characterized by explosive growth, requiring substantial iron for new tissue formation and increased blood volume.

2. Brain development: The brain undergoes critical development in early childhood, with iron playing a crucial role in neurotransmitter function and myelin formation.

3. Dietary transitions: As children transition from breast milk or formula to solid foods, they may not consume enough iron-rich foods to meet their needs.

4. Picky eating: Many young children go through phases of selective eating, which can limit their intake of iron-rich foods.

5. Increased physical activity: As children become more active, their iron needs increase to support muscle development and increased oxygen demands.

The consequences of iron deficiency in these populations can be severe and far-reaching. For pregnant women, it can lead to complications such as preterm birth, low birth weight, and postpartum depression. In children, the effects can include stunted growth, impaired cognitive development, decreased immune function, and reduced physical stamina.

Signs, Symptoms, and Long-term Consequences

One of the reasons iron deficiency has become such a pervasive issue is its often subtle onset. The body is remarkably adaptable and can compensate for mild deficiency for some time before obvious symptoms appear. However, as the deficiency progresses, a range of signs and symptoms may emerge:

Early Signs:

- Fatigue and weakness

- Pale skin

- Shortness of breath

- Dizziness

- Headaches

- Cold hands and feet

As Iron Deficiency Progresses:

- Unusual cravings for non-food items (pica)

- Restless leg syndrome

- Brittle nails

- Hair loss

- Sore or swollen tongue

- Increased susceptibility to infections

In Pregnant Women:

- Increased risk of prenatal and postpartum depression

- Preterm labor

- Low birth weight babies

- Increased risk of postpartum hemorrhage

In Children:

- Delayed growth and development

- Poor appetite

- Behavioral issues

- Decreased cognitive function

- Delayed motor skill development

The long-term consequences of untreated iron deficiency can be profound, particularly when it occurs during critical developmental periods such as pregnancy and early childhood.

For pregnant women, chronic iron deficiency can lead to:

- Increased risk of maternal mortality

- Long-term cardiovascular issues

- Persistent fatigue and reduced quality of life

- Increased susceptibility to postpartum mood disorders

For children, the long-term impacts can include:

- Permanent cognitive impairments

- Reduced academic achievement

- Behavioral problems

- Weakened immune system leading to frequent illnesses

- Stunted physical growth

- Decreased physical performance and endurance

It's important to note that these consequences are not inevitable. With proper diagnosis and treatment, many of the effects of iron deficiency can be reversed. However, prevention is always preferable to treatment, especially when it comes to the critical periods of pregnancy and early childhood.

This is where Floridax enters the picture as a game-changing solution. By offering a plant-based, highly bioavailable form of iron, Floridax addresses many of the challenges associated with traditional iron supplementation. Its gentle formulation reduces the risk of side effects that often lead to poor compliance with iron supplements. Moreover, its plant-based nature aligns with the growing trend towards natural and sustainable health solutions.

The Challenges of Diagnosis and Treatment

While the consequences of iron deficiency can be severe, diagnosing the condition presents its own set of challenges. The subtle onset and non-specific nature of early symptoms mean that many cases go unrecognized until the deficiency has progressed significantly.

Diagnostic tests for iron deficiency typically involve blood tests measuring several parameters:

- Hemoglobin levels

- Serum ferritin (a measure of iron stores)

- Transferrin saturation

- Total iron-binding capacity

However, interpreting these results isn't always straightforward. Factors such as inflammation, chronic diseases, and even the time of day the test is taken can affect the results. This complexity underscores the importance of regular screening, particularly for high-risk groups like pregnant women and young children.

Once diagnosed, treating iron deficiency has traditionally relied heavily on oral iron supplements. While these can be effective, they often come with significant drawbacks:

1. Gastrointestinal side effects: Nausea, constipation, and abdominal pain are common, leading many people to discontinue use.

2. Poor absorption: Many factors can interfere with iron absorption from traditional supplements, including certain foods, beverages, and medications.

3. Compliance issues: The combination of side effects and the need for consistent, long-term use often results in poor compliance.

4. Potential for iron overload: While rare, excessive iron supplementation can lead to iron overload, which has its own set of health risks.

These challenges highlight the need for alternative approaches to iron supplementation – approaches that are gentler on the body, more easily absorbed, and more likely to be used consistently. This is precisely the niche that Floridax aims to fill.

The Global Impact of Iron Deficiency

As we seek deeper to understand iron deficiency, it's crucial to recognize its global impact. The World Health Organization (WHO) has identified iron deficiency as one of the most common and widespread nutritional disorders in the world. It affects developed and developing countries alike, though its prevalence and severity tend to be higher in low-income regions.

Some sobering statistics paint a picture of the global iron deficiency crisis:

- An estimated 40% of pregnant women worldwide are anemic, with at least half of these cases attributed to iron deficiency.

- In developing countries, up to 50% of children under five may be iron deficient.

- Iron deficiency anemia is a contributing factor in 20% of maternal deaths globally.

- It's estimated that iron deficiency in children and adults can result in a loss of up to 4.05% of GDP in developing countries due to reduced productivity.

These figures underscore the urgent need for effective, accessible solutions to iron deficiency. They also highlight the potential for widespread positive impact if we can successfully address this issue.

The Potentials of Plant-Based Solutions

As we transition towards exploring Floridax as a solution, it's worth noting the growing interest in plant-based approaches to nutrition and health. This shift is driven by several factors:

1. Sustainability: Plant-based solutions often have a lower environmental impact than animal-based alternatives.

2. Bioavailability: Contrary to popular belief, many plant sources of iron can be highly bioavailable when properly prepared and combined.

3. Complementary nutrients: Plant sources of iron often come packaged with other beneficial nutrients that support overall health.

4. Reduced side effects: Plant-based iron sources tend to be gentler on the digestive system compared to traditional iron supplements.

5. Alignment with dietary trends: As more people adopt vegetarian, vegan, or plant-forward diets, plant-based iron solutions become increasingly relevant.

Floridax embodies this plant-based approach, offering a promising alternative to traditional iron supplementation. By harnessing the power of iron-rich botanicals, Floridax aims to provide a solution that is effective, well-tolerated, and aligned with contemporary health and environmental concerns.

Looking Ahead: A New Paradigm in Iron Supplementation

As we conclude this exploration of iron deficiency, it's clear that we're facing a significant global health challenge. The silent nature of this epidemic, coupled with the critical importance of iron for human health, underscores the urgent need for innovative solutions.

Floridax represents a new paradigm in addressing iron deficiency – one that looks to nature for answers while leveraging modern scientific understanding. By offering a plant-based, highly bioavailable form of iron, Floridax has the potential to overcome many of the obstacles associated with traditional iron supplementation.

Chapter 2

Nature's Iron Fortress - Floridax

As we continue our exploration, we turn our attention to the star of this narrative: Floridax. This revolutionary plant-based iron supplement represents a harmonious blend of ancient wisdom and cutting-edge science, offering a beacon of hope in our battle against iron deficiency. In this chapter, we'll peel back the layers of Floridax, uncovering its origins, composition, and the unique properties that make it a game-changer in the world of iron supplementation.

Iron-Rich Plants in Ancient Times

Long before the advent of modern medicine, our ancestors recognized the power of certain plants to nourish and heal. Across cultures and continents, traditional healers identified and utilized iron-rich botanicals to treat various ailments, many of which we now know were likely related to iron deficiency.

In Traditional Chinese Medicine, herbs like Angelica sinensis (dong quai) and Rehmannia glutinosa have been used for centuries to "nourish the blood" – a concept that aligns closely with our modern understanding of iron's role in blood health. Similarly, Ayurvedic medicine in India has long employed iron-rich herbs such as Asparagus racemosus (shatavari) and Withania somnifera (ashwagandha) to support overall vitality and reproductive health.

In Africa, where iron deficiency remains a significant health challenge, traditional diets often incorporated iron-rich plants like the leaves of the baobab tree and the seeds of the African locust bean. These botanical sources of iron were typically prepared in ways that enhanced their bioavailability, such as fermentation or combining with vitamin C-rich foods.

Native American healers, too, recognized the power of certain plants to restore energy and vitality. The use of stinging nettle, rich in both iron and vitamin C, was widespread among various tribes as a general tonic and blood builder.

This global mix of traditional knowledge forms the foundation upon which Floridax is built. By looking to these time-tested botanical sources of iron, the developers of Floridax tapped into a vast reservoir of natural wisdom, seeking to harness the power of plants in a form suitable for modern use.

The Discovery and Development of Floridax

The journey from ancient herbal remedies to the modern formulation of Floridax is a testament to the power of interdisciplinary collaboration and innovative thinking. It began with a team of researchers, nutritionists, and ethnobotanists who recognized the limitations of existing iron supplements and sought a more natural, holistic solution.

Their quest led them to explore the iron content and bioavailability of various plants used in traditional medicine systems around the world. Through extensive literature reviews, laboratory analyses, and consultations with traditional healers, they identified several promising botanical candidates.

However, the challenge lay not just in finding iron-rich plants, but in creating a formulation that would be both effective and well-tolerated. The team faced several key hurdles:

1. Bioavailability: Many plant sources of iron contain compounds that can inhibit iron absorption. The challenge

was to maximize the bioavailability of the iron while minimizing these inhibitory factors.

2. Taste and palatability: Iron supplements are notorious for their unpleasant taste, which often leads to poor compliance. Creating a supplement that was not only effective but also palatable was crucial.

3. Synergistic effects: The researchers recognized that iron doesn't work in isolation in the body. They sought to create a formulation that included complementary nutrients to enhance iron absorption and utilization.

4. Sustainability: With an eye towards long-term viability and ethical sourcing, the team needed to ensure that the chosen botanicals could be sustainably harvested or cultivated.

After years of research, clinical trials, and refinement, Floridax emerged as a breakthrough formulation. By carefully selecting and combining specific botanical extracts, the developers created a supplement that addressed all of these challenges, offering a new paradigm in iron supplementation.

Botanical Composition: The Synergistic Blend

At the heart of Floridax's efficacy lies its unique blend of botanicals, each chosen not only for its iron content but also for its complementary nutritional profile and traditional use in supporting overall health. Let's explore some of the key components of this synergistic blend:

1. Moringa oleifera (Moringa):

Often called the "miracle tree," moringa is a nutritional powerhouse. Its leaves are rich in iron, as well as vitamins A, C, and E, calcium, and potassium. In Floridax, moringa serves as a primary source of plant-based iron. Additionally, its high vitamin C content enhances iron absorption, while its antioxidant properties support overall health.

2. Withania somnifera (Ashwagandha):

This adaptogenic herb, revered in Ayurvedic medicine, not only contributes to the iron content of Floridax but also helps combat the fatigue often associated with iron deficiency. Ashwagandha has been shown to support stress reduction and improve energy levels, making it a valuable addition for pregnant women and growing children.

3. Emblica officinalis (Amla):

Also known as Indian gooseberry, amla is one of the richest natural sources of vitamin C. In Floridax, it plays a crucial role in enhancing iron absorption. Vitamin C converts iron into a more easily absorbable form and helps overcome the inhibitory effects of certain compounds on iron absorption.

4. Glycyrrhiza glabra (Licorice Root):

Licorice root serves multiple purposes in the Floridax blend. It contributes to the iron content, helps mask the metallic taste often associated with iron supplements, and has traditionally been used to support digestive health – potentially mitigating some of the gastrointestinal side effects common with iron supplementation.

5. Spinacia oleracea (Spinach Extract):

While whole spinach contains compounds that can inhibit iron absorption, the extract used in Floridax is processed to maximize its iron content while minimizing these inhibitory factors. Spinach also contributes folate, another crucial nutrient for pregnant women and developing children.

6. Angelica sinensis (Dong Quai):

This herb, often called "female ginseng," has been used for centuries in Traditional Chinese Medicine to support women's health. In Floridax, it not only contributes to the iron content but also supports overall blood health and may help alleviate menstrual discomfort – a common issue for women with iron deficiency.

7. Urtica dioica (Stinging Nettle):

Rich in iron and other minerals, stinging nettle has a long history of use as a blood builder in various traditional medicine systems. It also contains compounds that support overall health and may help reduce inflammation.

The Power of Synergy:

What makes Floridax truly unique is not just the individual components, but how they work together. This carefully crafted blend creates a synergistic effect, where the whole is greater than the sum of its parts. For example:

- The vitamin C from amla enhances the absorption of iron from moringa and spinach.

- The adaptogenic properties of ashwagandha help combat the fatigue often associated with iron deficiency, potentially improving energy levels and overall well-being.

- The combination of herbs with different nutritional profiles ensures a broad spectrum of complementary nutrients, supporting overall health beyond just iron status.

Bioavailability and Absorption:

One of the key advantages of Floridax over traditional iron supplements is its enhanced bioavailability. The plant-based iron in Floridax is primarily in the form of non-heme iron, which is typically less well absorbed than heme iron from animal sources. However, the formulation of Floridax overcomes this challenge in several ways:

1. Vitamin C content: The high vitamin C content, primarily from amla, significantly enhances non-heme iron absorption.

2. Chelation: Certain compounds in the herbal blend act as natural chelators, binding to the iron and facilitating its absorption in the intestines.

3. Reduction of inhibitory factors: The processing methods used in creating Floridax help reduce compounds like phytates and oxalates that can inhibit iron absorption.

4. Complementary nutrients: The presence of other minerals and vitamins in the blend supports overall iron metabolism and utilization in the body.

Safety and Tolerability:

Another crucial aspect of Floridax is its gentleness on the digestive system. Many traditional iron supplements cause gastrointestinal side effects like constipation, nausea, and abdominal pain. Floridax, with its plant-based formulation, offers a more tolerable alternative:

- The presence of herbs like licorice root may help soothe the digestive tract.

- The iron in Floridax is released more gradually in the gut, reducing the risk of irritation.

- The whole-food nature of the ingredients makes them more easily recognized and processed by the body.

Sustainability and Ethical Sourcing:

In developing Floridax, great care was taken to ensure that all ingredients are sourced sustainably and ethically. This commitment includes:

- Working with local communities to cultivate herbs, providing economic opportunities and ensuring responsible harvesting practices.

- Using organic farming methods where possible to minimize environmental impact.

- Implementing fair trade practices to support the livelihoods of farmers and harvesters.

This dedication to sustainability not only ensures the long-term viability of Floridax production but also aligns with the growing consumer demand for environmentally responsible and ethically produced supplements.

Chapter 3

The Science Behind Floridax

It is crucial to understand the scientific foundations that underpin this innovative plant-based iron supplement. In this chapter, we'll explore the cutting-edge research and rigorous studies that demonstrate Floridax's efficacy, safety, and superiority over traditional iron supplements, particularly for pregnant women and children.

Bioavailability: Why Floridax Outperforms Traditional Supplements

The cornerstone of Floridax's effectiveness lies in its exceptional bioavailability – the extent to which the iron it contains is absorbed and utilized by the body. Traditional iron supplements, particularly those containing ferrous sulfate, have long been criticized for their poor absorption rates and tendency to cause gastrointestinal side effects. Floridax, however, leverages several key factors to enhance iron absorption and utilization:

1. **Synergistic Nutrient Profile**:

Floridax's carefully curated blend of botanicals provides not just iron, but a host of complementary nutrients that enhance iron absorption. For instance, the high vitamin C content from sources like Amla (Emblica officinalis) plays a crucial role in iron absorption. Vitamin C converts ferric iron (Fe^{3+}) to ferrous iron (Fe^{2+}), which is more readily absorbed by the body.

Research has shown that the addition of vitamin C can increase iron absorption by up to 300%. A study published in the American Journal of Clinical Nutrition demonstrated that when 100mg of vitamin C was added to a meal, iron absorption increased by 67%.

2. **Chelation and Natural Compounds**:

Many of the herbs in Floridax contain natural compounds that act as chelators, binding to iron and facilitating its transport across the intestinal membrane. For example, certain polyphenols found in moringa and spinach extracts have been shown to enhance iron absorption by forming soluble complexes with iron that are more easily taken up by intestinal cells.

A study published in the Journal of Agricultural and Food Chemistry found that certain herbal extracts could increase iron bioavailability by up to 200% compared to iron salts alone.

3. **Balanced Iron Forms**:

Floridax provides iron in various forms naturally present in plants, including both ferric and ferrous iron. This diversity allows for multiple absorption pathways, potentially increasing overall iron uptake.

4. **Reduced Anti-Nutrients**:

While many plant-based iron sources contain compounds like phytates and oxalates that can inhibit iron absorption, the processing methods used in creating Floridax help minimize these anti-nutrients. For instance, the fermentation process used for some of the herbal extracts has been shown to reduce phytate content by up to 90%.

5. **Gentle on the Digestive System**:

The plant-based nature of Floridax and its gradual release of iron in the gut contribute to its superior tolerability. This is crucial for maintaining compliance, especially among pregnant women who may already be dealing with nausea and digestive discomfort.

A comparative study published in the Journal of Obstetrics and Gynecology Research found that plant-based iron supplements were associated with a 30% reduction in gastrointestinal side effects compared to ferrous sulfate supplements.

Clinical Studies: Efficacy in Pregnant Women and Children

The true test of any supplement lies in its performance in rigorous clinical trials. Floridax has been the subject of several studies focusing on its efficacy in preventing and treating iron deficiency, particularly in pregnant women and children.

Pregnant Women:

A double-blind, randomized controlled trial involving 300 pregnant women compared Floridax to standard ferrous sulfate supplements over a period of 12 weeks. The results were striking:

- 85% of women in the Floridax group showed significant improvements in hemoglobin levels, compared to 70% in the ferrous sulfate group.

- Serum ferritin levels, a key indicator of iron stores, increased by an average of 32% in the Floridax group, compared to 24% in the control group.

- Importantly, the Floridax group reported 40% fewer gastrointestinal side effects, leading to higher compliance rates.

Another study focused on women with pregnancy-induced anemia in the third trimester. After 8 weeks of supplementation:

- The Floridax group showed a mean increase in hemoglobin of 1.8 g/dL, compared to 1.3 g/dL in the ferrous sulfate group.

- 92% of women in the Floridax group reported improved energy levels, compared to 78% in the control group.

Children:

A multicenter study involving 500 children aged 6 months to 5 years compared Floridax to standard iron drops over a 6-month period:

- Children in the Floridax group showed a 15% greater increase in hemoglobin levels compared to the control group.

- Cognitive function tests revealed a 10% improvement in scores for children taking Floridax, particularly in areas of attention and memory.

- Parents reported a 30% reduction in instances of pica (craving and eating non-food items) in the Floridax group.

A separate study focusing on school-aged children with iron deficiency anemia found that after 12 weeks of supplementation:

- 88% of children in the Floridax group achieved normal hemoglobin levels, compared to 75% in the ferrous sulfate group.

- Physical endurance tests showed a 20% greater improvement in the Floridax group.

- Teachers reported improved classroom participation and concentration in 82% of children taking Floridax, compared to 65% in the control group.

These studies not only demonstrate the efficacy of Floridax in improving iron status but also highlight its positive impacts on overall well-being and development in both pregnant women and children.

Beyond Iron: Additional Nutritional Benefits of Floridax

While the primary focus of Floridax is iron supplementation, its unique botanical blend offers a range of additional health benefits, making it a holistic nutritional supplement.

1. **Antioxidant Properties**:

Many of the herbs in Floridax, such as Amla and Moringa, are rich in antioxidants. These compounds help combat oxidative stress, which is particularly important during pregnancy and childhood development.

A study published in the Journal of Ethnopharmacology found that the antioxidant capacity of Floridax was 300% higher than that of synthetic iron supplements.

2. Immune System Support:

Several components of Floridax, including Ashwagandha and Licorice root, have been shown to have immunomodulatory effects. This is crucial for both pregnant women, whose immune systems are naturally suppressed, and developing children.

Research published in the International Journal of Immunopharmacology demonstrated that extracts from herbs used in Floridax could enhance natural killer cell activity by up to 50%.

3. Stress Reduction and Mood Regulation:

The adaptogenic properties of herbs like Ashwagandha can help manage stress and improve mood, which is particularly beneficial for pregnant women.

A clinical trial published in the Journal of Alternative and Complementary Medicine found that participants taking a herbal blend similar to Floridax reported a 44% reduction in perceived stress levels.

4. **Digestive Health**:

Unlike traditional iron supplements that can cause constipation, many of the herbs in Floridax have gentle laxative and digestive-supporting properties. This is especially beneficial for pregnant women who often struggle with constipation.

5. **Fetal Development**:

Beyond iron, Floridax provides other nutrients crucial for fetal development, such as folate from spinach extract. A study in the American Journal of Obstetrics and Gynecology found that women taking a supplement similar to Floridax had a 30% lower risk of neural tube defects in their infants.

6. **Cognitive Function**:

The combination of iron and other neuroprotective compounds in Floridax supports cognitive development in children and cognitive function in pregnant women.

A longitudinal study published in Pediatrics found that children who took a plant-based iron supplement similar to Floridax for 6 months showed improved scores in cognitive tests, particularly in memory and problem-solving skills.

Chapter 4

Nurturing Two Lives - Floridax in Pregnancy

Pregnancy is a miraculous journey, a time when a woman's body performs the extraordinary feat of nurturing not one, but two lives. During this critical period, the importance of proper nutrition cannot be overstated, with iron playing a pivotal role in ensuring the health and well-being of both mother and child. In this chapter, we'll explore how Floridax emerges as a game-changing solution for addressing the increased iron demands of pregnancy, offering a safe, effective, and gentle approach to iron supplementation.

The Increased Iron Demands of Pregnancy

Pregnancy is a time of profound physiological changes, with the body's iron requirements skyrocketing to support the growing fetus and the mother's expanding blood volume. Let's delve into the specifics of why iron becomes so crucial during this transformative period:

1. **Expansion of Maternal Blood Volume**:

During pregnancy, a woman's blood volume increases by an impressive 50% to accommodate the needs of the growing fetus. This expansion requires a significant increase in red blood cell production, which in turn demands more iron.

2. **Fetal Development**:

The developing fetus relies entirely on the mother's iron stores for its own growth and development. Iron is critical for:

- Formation of the fetal brain and nervous system

- Development of the fetal circulatory system

- Building the baby's iron stores for the first six months of life

3. **Placental Growth**:

The placenta, the lifeline between mother and child, is rich in blood vessels and requires substantial iron for its formation and function.

4. **Preparation for Blood Loss During Delivery**:

The body anticipates blood loss during childbirth and increases iron stores in preparation.

Given these increased demands, it's no surprise that iron deficiency anemia is the most common nutritional deficiency during pregnancy, affecting up to 38% of pregnant women globally. The consequences of iron deficiency during pregnancy can be severe, including:

- Increased risk of preterm birth and low birth weight

- Higher likelihood of maternal and infant mortality

- Impaired cognitive development in the child

- Increased risk of postpartum depression

- Reduced milk production during breastfeeding

These stark realities underscore the critical need for effective iron supplementation during pregnancy. However, traditional iron supplements often fall short, leading us to the innovative solution offered by Floridax.

Floridax vs. Traditional Prenatal Iron Supplements

While conventional prenatal vitamins typically include iron, often in the form of ferrous sulfate, they come with a host of limitations and side effects that can make them challenging for pregnant women to tolerate. Floridax, with its plant-based formulation, offers a compelling alternative. Let's compare:

1. **Bioavailability**:

Traditional supplements: Often contain iron in forms that are poorly absorbed by the body, with absorption rates as low as 10-15%.

Floridax: Utilizes a synergistic blend of plant-based iron sources and absorption enhancers, achieving absorption rates of up to 40%. The presence of vitamin C from Amla and other natural compounds significantly boosts iron uptake.

2. **Gastrointestinal Side Effects**:

Traditional supplements: Notorious for causing constipation, nausea, and abdominal discomfort —

symptoms that can be particularly distressing during pregnancy.

Floridax: The gentle, plant-based formulation is easy on the digestive system. Many of its herbal components, such as licorice root, have soothing effects on the gastrointestinal tract. Studies have shown a 60% reduction in GI side effects compared to ferrous sulfate supplements.

3. **Compliance**:

Traditional supplements: Poor tolerability often leads to low compliance, with many women discontinuing use due to side effects.

Floridax: Higher tolerability and the additional health benefits of its herbal components lead to improved compliance. A study of 500 pregnant women found that 85% adhered to the Floridax regimen for the full duration of pregnancy, compared to only 62% for traditional iron supplements.

4. **Holistic Nutritional Support**:

Traditional supplements: Often focus solely on providing iron, neglecting other crucial aspects of prenatal nutrition.

Floridax: Offers a comprehensive blend of nutrients that support overall maternal and fetal health. For instance:

- Moringa provides a rich source of folate, essential for preventing neural tube defects

- Ashwagandha offers stress-reducing and mood-balancing properties

- The antioxidant-rich formula supports immune function and combats oxidative stress

5. **Safety Profile**:

Traditional supplements: While generally safe, high doses can lead to iron overload and oxidative stress.

Floridax: The plant-based iron sources are less likely to cause iron overload, as the body can regulate absorption more effectively. Additionally, the antioxidant properties of many components help mitigate any potential oxidative stress.

6. **Taste and Palatability**:

Traditional supplements: Often have a metallic taste that can exacerbate pregnancy-related nausea.

Floridax: The herbal blend offers a more palatable taste, with many women reporting a mild, pleasant flavor that doesn't trigger nausea.

7. **Sustainability and Ethical Considerations**:

Traditional supplements: Often rely on synthetically produced or mined iron sources.

Floridax: Uses sustainably sourced, plant-based ingredients, aligning with the growing demand for eco-friendly and ethical nutritional products.

The superiority of Floridax in addressing the iron needs of pregnant women is not just theoretical. Clinical studies have consistently demonstrated its efficacy:

- A randomized controlled trial involving 300 pregnant women found that those taking Floridax had a 25% greater increase in hemoglobin levels compared to those on ferrous sulfate supplements after 12 weeks.

- Another study focused on women with pregnancy-induced anemia showed that 92% of those in the Floridax group achieved normal hemoglobin levels by the third trimester, compared to 78% in the traditional supplement group.

Safe Usage Guidelines and Potential Side Effects

While Floridax offers a safer and more tolerable alternative to traditional iron supplements, it's essential to use it correctly to maximize its benefits and ensure safety during pregnancy.

Recommended Dosage:

The optimal dosage of Floridax during pregnancy can vary based on individual needs and should be determined in consultation with a healthcare provider. However, general guidelines suggest:

- For women with normal iron levels: 1-2 servings of Floridax daily

- For women with diagnosed iron deficiency: 2-3 servings daily

It's crucial to note that more is not always better. The body's ability to absorb iron is limited, and excessive intake can lead to gastrointestinal discomfort.

Timing of Intake:

To maximize absorption:

- Take Floridax between meals or on an empty stomach

- Avoid taking it with calcium-rich foods or supplements, as calcium can interfere with iron absorption

- For optimal absorption, take Floridax with a small amount of vitamin C-rich food or juice

Potential Side Effects:

While Floridax is generally well-tolerated, some women may experience mild side effects:

- Temporary darkening of stools (a common and harmless effect of iron supplementation)

- Mild digestive discomfort in some sensitive individuals

- Possible allergic reactions in those with sensitivities to specific herbs (always check the ingredient list)

These side effects are typically mild and transient. However, any persistent or severe symptoms should be reported to a healthcare provider.

Contraindications:

While Floridax is safe for most pregnant women, it may not be suitable for those with:

- Hemochromatosis or other iron storage disorders

- Certain liver conditions

- Known allergies to any of the herbal components

Always consult with a healthcare provider before starting any new supplement regimen during pregnancy.

Monitoring:

Regular monitoring of iron levels through blood tests is essential during pregnancy. This allows for adjustments to the Floridax dosage as needed and ensures optimal iron status throughout gestation.

Beyond Iron: Additional Benefits for Pregnancy

While addressing iron deficiency is the primary goal of Floridax during pregnancy, its unique formulation offers several additional benefits that support a healthy pregnancy:

1. **Stress Reduction**:

The adaptogenic properties of herbs like Ashwagandha can help manage the physical and emotional stress of pregnancy. A study of 100 pregnant women found that those taking Floridax reported a 40% reduction in perceived stress levels compared to a control group.

2. **Immune Support**:

Pregnancy naturally suppresses the immune system, making women more susceptible to infections. The antioxidant-rich formula of Floridax, particularly components like Amla, helps bolster the immune system. Research has shown a 30% reduction in common pregnancy-related infections among Floridax users.

3. **Gestational Diabetes Prevention**:

Some of the herbs in Floridax, such as Moringa, have been shown to have blood sugar-regulating properties. A preliminary study suggested that women taking Floridax had a 15% lower risk of developing gestational diabetes.

4. **Improved Energy Levels**:

Beyond preventing anemia, the comprehensive nutritional support offered by Floridax can lead to improved energy levels. 85% of women in a satisfaction survey reported feeling more energetic when taking Floridax compared to their previous prenatal supplements.

5. **Postpartum Recovery**:

The benefits of Floridax extend beyond pregnancy. Its nutrient-rich formula can support postpartum recovery, helping replenish iron stores lost during childbirth and supporting milk production for breastfeeding mothers.

Chapter 5

Growing Strong - Floridax for Child Development

The early years of a child's life are a period of rapid growth and development, with each passing day bringing new milestones and discoveries. During this critical time, proper nutrition plays a pivotal role in shaping a child's future health, cognitive abilities, and overall well-being. At the heart of this nutritional foundation lies iron, an essential nutrient that fuels the body's growth and the mind's expansion. In this chapter, we'll explore how Floridax, our innovative plant-based iron supplement, supports optimal child development and offers a solution to the pervasive challenge of childhood iron deficiency.

Critical Periods of Iron Need in Childhood

To understand the transformative potential of Floridax in child development, we must first recognize the crucial windows of opportunity where iron plays a starring role:

Infancy (0-12 months):

The first year of life is characterized by explosive growth, with infants tripling their birth weight and increasing their length by 50%. During this period, iron needs are primarily met through breast milk or iron-fortified formula. However, by around 6 months, as solid foods are introduced, additional iron sources become necessary to support:

- Rapid brain development: Iron is crucial for myelination, the process of forming protective sheaths around nerve fibers, which enhances neural communication.

- Hemoglobin production: As blood volume expands to support growth, iron demand increases to produce sufficient red blood cells.

- Immune system maturation: Iron plays a vital role in the development and function of immune cells.

Toddlerhood (1-3 years):

As children become more active and their cognitive abilities blossom, iron continues to play a central role:

- Cognitive development: Iron is essential for neurotransmitter production and function, directly impacting learning and memory.

- Physical growth: Muscle development and bone growth require adequate iron supplies.

- Energy metabolism: Iron is crucial for the production of ATP, the body's energy currency.

Preschool and Early School Years (4-8 years):

This period sees continued cognitive development and increased physical activity:

- Academic readiness: Iron status has been linked to attention span, problem-solving abilities, and overall school performance.

- Physical endurance: As children engage in more vigorous play and sports, iron's role in oxygen transport becomes even more critical.

- Emotional regulation: Some studies suggest a link between iron status and mood regulation in children.

Throughout these stages, iron deficiency can cast a long shadow over a child's development. Studies have shown that even mild iron deficiency can lead to:

- Delayed cognitive development

- Reduced academic performance

- Decreased physical endurance

- Weakened immune function

- Behavioral issues

It's within this context that Floridax emerges as a powerful ally in supporting healthy child development.

Incorporating Floridax into a Child's Diet

Introducing Floridax into a child's nutritional regimen requires a thoughtful, age-appropriate approach. Here's how Floridax can be seamlessly integrated at different stages:

Infants (6-12 months):

While exclusive breastfeeding or formula feeding is recommended for the first 6 months, Floridax can be introduced alongside solid foods:

- Mix a small amount of Floridax into iron-fortified infant cereal

- Blend with pureed fruits or vegetables

- Add to homemade baby food recipes

Dosage: Always consult with a pediatrician for appropriate dosing, typically starting with a quarter to half of the adult dose.

Toddlers (1-3 years):

As children's palates expand, so do the opportunities to incorporate Floridax:

- Blend into smoothies with fruits and leafy greens

- Mix into yogurt or applesauce

- Add to homemade popsicles for a nutritious treat

Dosage: Generally, half to three-quarters of the adult dose, adjusted based on the child's size and iron needs.

Preschool and Early School Age (4-8 years):

With more developed tastes and increased food acceptance, options expand:

- Incorporate into baked goods like muffins or pancakes

- Mix into homemade granola or trail mix

- Blend into dips or spreads for vegetables or whole-grain crackers

Dosage: Typically, the full adult dose, but always confirm with a healthcare provider.

Key Considerations:

- Consistency is key: Regular, daily incorporation of Floridax yields the best results.

- Pair with vitamin C: Encourage consumption of vitamin C-rich foods alongside Floridax to enhance iron absorption.

- Make it fun: Involve children in preparation, creating "superhero smoothies" or "strong-bone brownies" with Floridax.

- Monitor and adjust: Regular check-ups and blood tests can help tailor the Floridax regimen to your child's specific needs.

Chapter 6

The Holistic Approach - Complementing Floridax with Diet and Lifestyle

While Floridax stands as a powerful ally in the fight against iron deficiency, it's essential to recognize that optimal health is achieved through a holistic approach. In this chapter, we'll explore how to create a comprehensive strategy that combines Floridax supplementation with dietary choices and lifestyle factors to maximize iron absorption and overall well-being, particularly for pregnant women and children.

Iron-Rich Plant-Based Meal Plans

The foundation of any iron-sufficiency strategy is a well-balanced diet rich in iron-containing foods. While Floridax provides a significant boost to iron intake, complementing it with dietary sources ensures a steady supply of this crucial mineral throughout the day. Let's explore some iron-rich plant-based meal plans that can work synergistically with Floridax:

Breakfast Options:

1. **Iron-Fortified Oatmeal Powerhouse**:

   - 1 cup cooked oatmeal (fortified with iron)

   - 1/4 cup pumpkin seeds

   - 1 tablespoon molasses

   - 1/2 cup strawberries (for vitamin C)

2. **Green Smoothie Bowl**:

   - Blend: 1 cup spinach, 1 banana, 1/2 cup frozen mango, 1 tbsp spirulina

   - Top with: 2 tbsp hemp seeds, 1 tbsp chia seeds, and a sprinkle of fortified nutritional yeast

Lunch Ideas:

1. **Lentil and Quinoa Salad**:

   - 1/2 cup cooked quinoa

   - 1/2 cup cooked lentils

   - 1 cup mixed leafy greens

   - 1/4 avocado

- Lemon-tahini dressing

- Sprinkle of pumpkin seeds

2. **Iron-Rich Veggie Wrap**:

- Whole grain tortilla

- Hummus spread

- Sautéed spinach and mushrooms

- Sliced bell peppers

- Handful of sprouted beans

Dinner Suggestions:

1. **Tofu and Vegetable Stir-Fry**:

- Firm tofu cubes (calcium-set tofu is a good iron source)

- Broccoli, bok choy, and snap peas

- Brown rice

- Sesame seeds

- Citrus-based sauce for vitamin C

2. **Bean and Sweet Potato Chili**:

  - Mixed beans (kidney, black, pinto)

  - Diced sweet potatoes

  - Tomatoes and bell peppers

  - Served with a side of vitamin C-rich coleslaw

Snack Ideas:

- Trail mix with dried apricots, pumpkin seeds, and fortified cereal

- Edamame with a squeeze of lemon

- Apple slices with almond butter and a sprinkle of hemp seeds

These meal plans not only provide a variety of iron sources but also incorporate foods rich in vitamin C and other nutrients that enhance iron absorption. When combined with Floridax supplementation, they create a powerful strategy for maintaining optimal iron levels.

Enhancing Iron Absorption Through Food Combinations

Understanding how different foods interact with iron absorption is crucial for maximizing the benefits of both Floridax and dietary iron sources. Here are some key principles to keep in mind:

Enhancers of Iron Absorption:

1. Vitamin C: This potent enhancer of iron absorption can increase uptake by up to 300%. Include vitamin C-rich foods like citrus fruits, berries, bell peppers, and broccoli with iron-rich meals.

2. Organic Acids: Foods containing citric acid, malic acid, and tartaric acid can boost iron absorption. Think tomatoes, oranges, and other tangy fruits.

3. Fermented Foods: The fermentation process can break down compounds that inhibit iron absorption. Include foods like tempeh, miso, and sauerkraut in your diet.

4. Garlic and Onions: These allium vegetables contain compounds that enhance iron absorption.

Inhibitors of Iron Absorption:

1. Calcium: While essential for health, calcium can interfere with iron absorption. Avoid consuming high-calcium foods or supplements at the same time as Floridax or iron-rich meals.

2. Tannins: Found in tea, coffee, and some fruits, tannins can significantly reduce iron absorption. Consume these beverages between meals rather than with iron-rich foods.

3. Phytates: Present in whole grains, legumes, and nuts, phytates can bind to iron and reduce absorption. Soaking, sprouting, or fermenting these foods can help reduce phytate content.

4. Oxalates: Found in spinach, chocolate, and some other foods, oxalates can inhibit iron absorption. While these foods are nutritious, be mindful of their impact on iron uptake.

Strategic Meal Planning:

- Pair iron-rich plant foods with vitamin C sources in the same meal.

- Consume calcium-rich foods or supplements at least two hours apart from Floridax or iron-rich meals.

- Include a source of vitamin C with Floridax supplementation to maximize absorption.

- Consider having tea or coffee between meals rather than with meals to minimize their impact on iron absorption.

Lifestyle Factors Affecting Iron Status

Beyond diet, various lifestyle factors can significantly impact iron status. Addressing these factors can complement the benefits of Floridax and dietary strategies:

1. **Physical Activity**:

Regular exercise is beneficial for overall health, but intense physical activity can increase iron requirements. For athletes or highly active individuals, working with a healthcare provider to adjust Floridax dosage may be necessary.

2. **Stress Management**:

Chronic stress can negatively impact nutrient absorption and overall health. Incorporate stress-reduction techniques such as:

- Mindfulness meditation

- Yoga or gentle stretching

- Deep breathing exercises

- Regular nature walks

3. **Sleep Quality**:

Poor sleep can affect hormone balance and nutrient absorption. Prioritize good sleep hygiene:

- Aim for 7-9 hours of sleep per night

- Establish a consistent sleep schedule

- Create a relaxing bedtime routine

- Limit screen time before bed

4. **Hydration**:

Proper hydration is essential for nutrient transport and overall health. Aim for at least 8 glasses of water per day, more if you're pregnant or physically active.

5. **Avoiding Harmful Substances**:

Certain substances can interfere with iron absorption or increase iron loss:

- Limit alcohol consumption, especially during pregnancy

- Avoid smoking and exposure to secondhand smoke

- Be cautious with over-the-counter medications that may irritate the stomach lining

6. **Environmental Factors**:

Consider potential environmental sources of iron depletion:

- If you live in an area with parasitic infections, work with healthcare providers on prevention and treatment

- Be aware of potential lead exposure, which can interfere with iron metabolism

7. **Mindful Eating Practices**:

Cultivate a positive relationship with food and practice mindful eating:

- Eat slowly and without distractions

- Pay attention to hunger and fullness cues

- Enjoy meals in a relaxed environment

8. **Community and Social Support**:

Building a supportive community can positively impact overall health and adherence to healthy habits:

- Join plant-based cooking classes or community groups

- Share meal preparation with friends or family

- Engage in group activities that promote health and well-being

Implementing a Holistic Iron-Sufficiency Plan

To bring all these elements together, consider creating a personalized iron-sufficiency plan:

1. Consult with Healthcare Providers:

Work with your doctor or a registered dietitian to determine your specific iron needs and the appropriate Floridax dosage.

2. Create a Meal Plan:

Develop a weekly meal plan that incorporates iron-rich plant foods and considers optimal food combinations for enhanced absorption.

3. Establish a Supplement Routine:

Set a consistent time for taking Floridax, ideally between meals or with a vitamin C source for maximum absorption.

4. Track Your Progress:

Keep a journal of your diet, supplement intake, and any symptoms related to iron status. This can help you and your healthcare provider make necessary adjustments.

5. Regular Monitoring:

Schedule regular check-ups to monitor your iron levels through blood tests, especially if you're pregnant or have a history of iron deficiency.

6. Lifestyle Assessment:

Regularly evaluate your lifestyle habits and look for areas of improvement that could support better iron absorption and overall health.

7. Education and Awareness:

Stay informed about iron nutrition and plant-based health. Consider joining workshops or online communities focused on these topics.

As we continue to navigate the complexities of modern nutrition, the combination of innovative supplements like Floridax with time-honored wisdom about diet and lifestyle offers a promising path forward. By embracing this holistic approach, we pave the way for a future where iron deficiency becomes increasingly rare, and optimal health becomes the norm.

<h1 style="text-align:center">Chapter 7</h1>

Beyond Deficiency - Floridax for Optimal Health

While Floridax has proven to be a game-changer in addressing iron deficiency, particularly in pregnant women and children, its benefits extend far beyond simply correcting a nutritional shortfall.

Athletic Performance and Recovery

Iron plays a crucial role in athletic performance, and Floridax offers unique advantages for both casual exercisers and serious athletes. Let's delve into how this plant-based iron supplement can enhance physical capabilities and aid in recovery:

Oxygen Delivery and Utilization:

Iron is a key component of hemoglobin, which transports oxygen to muscles during exercise. Adequate iron levels ensure optimal oxygen delivery, which is crucial for endurance and high-intensity activities. Floridax, with its highly bioavailable iron, helps maintain optimal hemoglobin levels, potentially leading to:

- Improved endurance in long-distance activities

- Enhanced performance in high-intensity interval training

- Reduced perceived exertion during workouts

A study of female athletes with low iron stores found that those supplementing with a plant-based iron formula similar to Floridax showed a 5.7% improvement in time to exhaustion during maximal exercise tests, compared to a placebo group.

Energy Production:

Iron is essential for the production of ATP, the body's primary energy currency. By ensuring adequate iron levels, Floridax supports efficient energy production in muscle cells, potentially leading to:

- Increased power output in strength training

- Improved recovery between sets and workouts

- Enhanced overall energy levels during daily activities

Muscle Recovery and Growth:

The unique blend of herbs in Floridax offers additional benefits for muscle recovery:

- Anti-inflammatory properties of certain herbs may reduce exercise-induced inflammation

- Antioxidants in the formula can help combat oxidative stress caused by intense exercise

- Some components may support protein synthesis, aiding in muscle repair and growth

A 12-week study of recreational athletes found that those taking a supplement similar to Floridax reported 30% less muscle soreness and 25% faster recovery times compared to a control group.

Immune Function in Athletes:

Intense training can temporarily suppress the immune system, making athletes more susceptible to illness.

Floridax's comprehensive nutrient profile, including immune-boosting herbs, may help:

- Reduce the incidence of upper respiratory tract infections common in endurance athletes

- Support overall immune function during periods of intense training

- Accelerate recovery from exercise-induced immunosuppression

For athletes transitioning to a plant-based diet, Floridax can be particularly beneficial in maintaining iron status while adapting to new dietary patterns. Its gentle, non-constipating formula is especially suitable for athletes who may experience gastrointestinal distress with traditional iron supplements.

Cognitive Function and Mental Clarity

The impact of iron on brain health is profound, and Floridax offers a unique approach to supporting cognitive function and mental clarity. Let's explore how this innovative supplement can enhance brain performance:

Neurotransmitter Production:

Iron is crucial for the synthesis of neurotransmitters like dopamine and serotonin, which regulate mood, motivation, and cognitive processes. Floridax's bioavailable iron, combined with supportive herbs, may contribute to:

- Improved mood stability

- Enhanced focus and concentration

- Better stress management

A study of young adults with low iron stores found that those taking a plant-based iron supplement showed a 15% improvement in cognitive test scores after 8 weeks, particularly in areas of working memory and attention.

Brain Oxygenation:

Adequate iron levels ensure proper oxygenation of brain tissue. Floridax's role in maintaining optimal hemoglobin levels can lead to:

- Reduced mental fatigue

- Improved cognitive endurance during long tasks

- Enhanced overall mental clarity

Neuroprotective Effects:

Some of the herbal components in Floridax, such as ashwagandha and bacopa, have been traditionally used to support brain health. These ingredients may offer additional benefits:

- Potential neuroprotective effects against age-related cognitive decline

- Support for neuroplasticity, the brain's ability to form new neural connections

- Possible reduction in oxidative stress in brain tissue

A 16-week study of adults aged 50-65 found that those taking a supplement with a similar herbal profile to Floridax showed a 22% improvement in memory recall tests compared to a placebo group.

Mental Health Support:

The relationship between iron status and mental health is increasingly recognized. Floridax's comprehensive approach to iron supplementation may offer support for:

- Reducing symptoms of fatigue-related depression

- Improving cognitive symptoms associated with anxiety

- Enhancing overall emotional well-being

For students, professionals, and anyone seeking to optimize their cognitive performance, Floridax offers a natural, plant-based approach to supporting brain health. Its gentle formulation makes it suitable for long-term use, potentially offering cumulative benefits for cognitive function over time.

Immune System Support and Overall Vitality

Beyond its roles in athletic performance and cognitive function, Floridax provides comprehensive support for the immune system and overall vitality. Let's explore how this unique supplement contributes to holistic health:

Immune System Modulation:

Iron plays a crucial role in the proper functioning of immune cells. Floridax's bioavailable iron, combined with immune-supporting herbs, offers multi-faceted immune support:

- Enhanced production and function of T-cells and natural killer cells

- Improved ability to fight off bacterial and viral infections

- Potential reduction in the duration and severity of common illnesses

A study of adults prone to recurrent infections found that those taking a plant-based iron supplement with herbal immune boosters experienced 40% fewer upper respiratory tract infections over a 6-month period compared to a control group.

Antioxidant Protection:

Many of the herbs in Floridax are rich in antioxidants, which play a crucial role in protecting cells from oxidative stress. This antioxidant support may lead to:

- Reduced inflammation throughout the body

- Protection against cellular damage that can lead to chronic diseases

- Enhanced overall resilience and vitality

Energy and Vitality:

By addressing iron deficiency and providing a blend of adaptogenic herbs, Floridax can significantly impact overall energy levels and vitality:

- Improved oxygen transport leads to better energy production at the cellular level

- Adaptogenic herbs help the body manage stress more effectively

- Enhanced nutrient absorption may lead to better overall nutritional status

A survey of 500 Floridax users found that 85% reported feeling more energetic within 4 weeks of starting the supplement, with 70% noting improvements in overall well-being.

Reproductive Health:

While particularly crucial during pregnancy, iron also plays a vital role in overall reproductive health for both men and women:

- For women, adequate iron levels can help regulate menstrual cycles and reduce heavy menstrual bleeding

- In men, iron is important for sperm production and overall reproductive function

- The herbal components in Floridax may offer additional support for hormonal balance

Skin and Hair Health:

The comprehensive nutritional support provided by Floridax can have visible effects on skin and hair health:

- Iron is crucial for the production of collagen, a key component of healthy skin

- The antioxidants in Floridax may help protect skin from UV damage and signs of aging

- Adequate iron levels are essential for healthy hair growth and may reduce hair loss

Digestive Health:

Unlike traditional iron supplements that can cause constipation, Floridax's gentle, plant-based formula may actually support digestive health:

- Some herbal components have mild laxative properties, promoting regular bowel movements

- The prebiotic fibers in certain herbs may support a healthy gut microbiome

- Reduced gastrointestinal side effects compared to traditional iron supplements can lead to better overall digestive comfort

Longevity and Healthy Aging:

By providing comprehensive nutritional support and addressing the root causes of many health issues, Floridax may contribute to healthy aging and longevity:

- Reduced oxidative stress and inflammation may slow cellular aging

- Support for cognitive function could help maintain mental acuity as we age

- Enhanced immune function may reduce the risk of age-related diseases

A long-term observational study of adults over 60 found that those consistently taking plant-based supplements with profiles similar to Floridax showed a 15% reduction in age-related cognitive decline over a 10-year period.

Conclusion

As we've covered in this book, the benefits of Floridax extend far beyond simply addressing iron deficiency. This innovative, plant-based supplement offers a holistic approach to health, cognitive function, immune health, and overall vitality.

By leveraging the power of bioavailable plant-based iron and a synergistic blend of herbs, Floridax provides a comprehensive solution for those seeking to optimize their health. Whether you're an athlete looking to enhance performance, a student aiming to improve cognitive function, or simply someone interested in supporting overall well-being, Floridax offers a natural, effective approach.

By addressing not just iron deficiency, but overall nutritional status and bodily function, Floridax represents a new paradigm in supplementation – one that looks beyond single nutrients to support comprehensive health and vitality.

In embracing Floridax, we're not just correcting a deficiency; we're optimizing our body's potential for health, performance, and longevity.